ALL YOU WAN

Refl

VIJAYA KUMAR

New Dawn

NEW DAWN
An imprint of Sterling Publishers (P) Ltd.
A-59 Okhla Industrial Area, Phase-II,
New Delhi-110020.
Tel: 6916209, 6916165, 6912677, 6910050
Fax: 91-11-6331241 E-mail: ghai@nde.vsnl.net.in
www.sterlingpublishers.com

All You Wanted to Know About Reflexology
©2002, Sterling Publishers Private Limited
ISBN 81 207 2449 6

Published by Sterling Publishers Pvt. Ltd., New Delhi-110020.
Lasertypeset by Vikas Compographics, New Delhi-110020.
Printed at Sai Printers, New Delhi-110020.

Contents

- Bell's Palsy - Breast Cysts - Bronchitis
- Bursitis- Cancer - Catarrh - Chilblain
- Colitis - Coma - Conjunctivitis
- Constipation - Cough - Cramp - Cystitis
- Deafness - Depression - Dermatitis
- Diabetes - Diarrhoea - Earache - Eczema
- Emphysema - Epilepsy - Eye Strain
- Fibroids - Fibrositis - Flatulence - Frozen
Shoulder - Gallstones - Glaucoma - Goitre
- Gout - Haemorrhoid - Hay Fever
- Headaches - Heart Attack - Hepatitis
- Hernia - Hypertension - Hypoglycaemia
- Hypotension - Incontinence - Indigestion
- Infertility - Insomnia - Jaundice
- Kidney Stone - Knee Pain - Lumbago
- Mastitis - Ménière's Disease - Meningitis
- Menopause - Migraine - Multiple
Nephritis - Neuralgia - Ovarian Cysts
- Paralysis - Parkinson's Disease - Phlebitis
- Pleurisy - Premenstrual Tension
- Prostate Enlargement - Psoriasis
- Raynaud's Disease - Rheumatism
- Rhinitis - Sciatica - Sclerosis - Shingles
- Sinusitis - Spondylitis - Stroke - Tennis
Elbow - Tenosynovitis - Thrombosis
- Tinnitus - Tonsillitis - Toothache - Ulcers
- Varicose Veins - Vertigo

Introduction

Reflexology is a unique, complementary health modality, which involves massaging of all the areas of the feet mainly, using one's natural touch therapy, though at times reflexologists prefer to give their patient the option of massaging the hands too. Especially those who find it cumbersome to bend down to massage the foot continuously for ten minutes or more. Reflexes have an amazing potential for communicating, just like a telephone or a computer keyboard. And like for the keyboard, you must apply your touch to make the connection.

The main concept of reflexology is its effective balancing of the mind and body in a safe manner, and helping one to deal with the strains and stresses of everyday life. Explore this gift of natural touch, use it with vitality, and the rewards will amaze and fascinate you!

What is Reflexology?

- Reflexology is a form of treatment involving touch on the areas of the feet and hands, whereby the corresponding areas of the body get stimulated.
- These reflex areas are found on the soles, the top and the sides of the feet, as well as on the hands and ears.
- Massaging these reflex areas helps in balancing the mind and the body, and correcting those parts that are malfunctioning.

- Since the feet are more responsive than the hands, practitioners prefer to use the former for healing.
- The feet also provide a wider and larger area to be treated as compared with hands or ears.
- Since the feet are generally covered and protected by shoes and socks, or even slippers, they offer a more sensitive area than hands for the treatment.
- Hands can be used if one finds them more convenient.
- Reflexology, like the Chinese acupuncture, has energy lines

linking the hands and feet to various parts of the body.

- Stimulating the feet is a natural touch therapy that has been used for centuries.
- The feet that literally carry us through life, are often the most neglected parts of our body, and need the utmost care, as they are most vital for reflexology to work.
- Reflex areas are similar to push buttons that convey messages to the rest of the body.
- Unlike acupressure or acu-puncture, reflexology is more for giving and is very easy to learn.

- The reflex areas are quite wide and large, and once you know all about the body-foot relationship, you can navigate your body and then the foot, to use your touch.
- In these reflex areas, the affected parts of the body show up as tender spots.
- Once you get familiar with reflexing the feet, you may experiment with hands and outer ears.

Benefits of Reflexology

- Reflexology provides the ability to cope with the negative stresses of life.
- It unclogs the blockages of energy, resulting from stresses accumulating in the reflex areas.

- Once these energies are released, the cells benefit the most, for they get more energy from blood nutrients, more oxygen and a normal delivery of electrical impulses.
- Hence, by reflexing the feet, or hand or ears, you can help to normalise your body functions.
- Pain gets alleviated and you experience better health.
- With all the body parts finely tuned and relaxed, health becomes a symphony!
- Your resistance to diseases and ailments increases.

- As a self-help process, reflexology is easy to learn.
- It can be used to alleviate stress from chronic conditions.
- It helps the spirit and emotions to be light and positive.
- It steers your mental attitude towards sharpness and better focus.

Artificial and Natural Stimulants

- Commercially, there are a number of reflex tools for stimulating the feet.
- A reflex tool is anything you use to apply pressure to reflex areas, other than your own touch.
- The most notable among these tools are prayer and rosary beads,

providing comfort and relaxation to several people around the world.

- These beads, held in one hand and counted, one by one, between the index finger and the thumb, apply pressure between them, and the pituitary gland, which has connection with the fleshy part of the thumb, gets activated, thus reducing stress.

Rosary Beads

- Rolling feet on a ball stimulates the affected parts and brings relief to them.

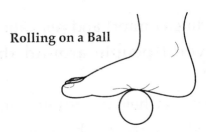

Rolling on a Ball

- Pressure can be applied using the edge of a stair, while holding on to something solid for support.

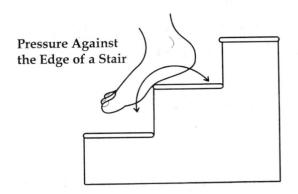

Pressure Against the Edge of a Stair

- Walking on smooth stones, sand, wet grass, etc. is beneficial because electromagnetic forces from the earth move into your body via your feet.

- Animals, who wear no footwear, benefit all the time!
- Apart from foot-rollers, there are rubber-spiked balls, mini-massagers, electric, vibrating pads, foot-baths, etc. that are commercially used for reflexology.

Examples of Rollers

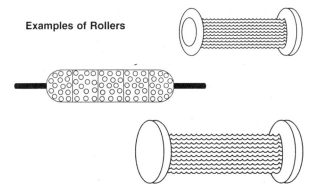

- Just remember that what tool might be very good for someone else may not be as good for you, since everybody has different sensitivities.
- Electric stimulating devices come with various speed or vibration settings.
- Those that are floor units with stimulating pads or roller balls under a soft cover make a general stimulus to the reflexes.
- The ones with rollers work the reflexes much deeper and more effectively.

Reflexes and the Body

- The body is divided into three parts to make the learning process easier.
- The reflexes on the *soles* of the feet are related to the main part, or torso, and the head.
- The reflexes on the *outside* of the feet are related to the sides of the body.
- The reflexes on the *inside edges* of the feet relate to the centre line of the body.
- The numbers in the two diagrams (*Main Body Divisions* and *Main Reflex Divisions*) correspond to each

17

Main Body Divisions

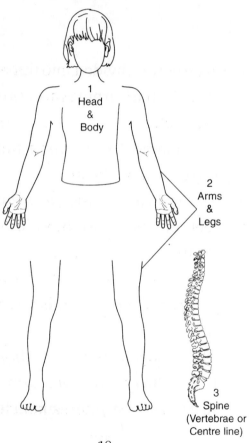

1
Head
&
Body

2
Arms
&
Legs

3
Spine
(Vertebrae or
Centre line)

Main Reflex Divisions

1
Soles of
the Feet

2
Outside of
the Feet

3
Inside of
the Feet

other, that is, the body numbers are related to the feet numbers.

- The toes are considered as the top part of the foot, and correspond to the top of the body, which is the head.

19

- Working from top to bottom, there are five main divisions of the body and feet as shown below:

Main (Horizontal) Division Areas

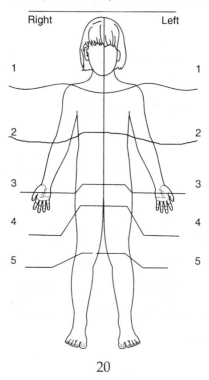

Main Reflex Areas

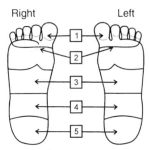

- The main divisions, then, are the head and neck, chest and shoulders, upper abdomen, lower abdomen and pelvic region.

- Next, the right foot is related to the right side of the body, whereas the left foot corresponds to the left side of the body.

- Let us take, for example, the lungs and the colon (large intestine). The diagram on the following page explains the concept of reflexology.

Example of Lung and Colon

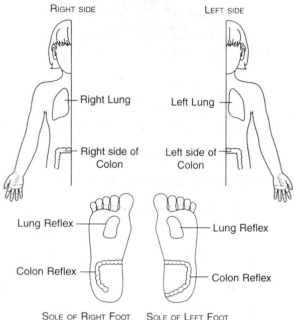

RIGHT SIDE

LEFT SIDE

Right Lung

Left Lung

Right side of Colon

Left side of Colon

Lung Reflex

Lung Reflex

Colon Reflex

Colon Reflex

SOLE OF RIGHT FOOT   SOLE OF LEFT FOOT

• Once you understand these divisions well, it will be easier to proceed to the next stage – getting to the correct reflex area of the foot.

- Exploring the area on the foot that corresponds to the area of the body is called navigating.

- Like latitudes and longitudes that are used for locating places on a map, the body, too, can be divided horizontally and vertically, from head down to the fingers, and from head down to the toes.

- The imbalance in the body can be traced along its zone to a reflex in the same zone of the foot or hand.

- Like the five horizontal divisions, the body can also be divided into five vertical zones, relating to each foot and each hand.

Main (Vertical) Division Areas

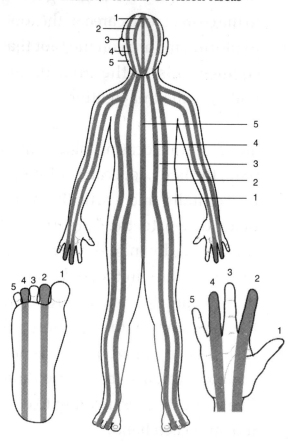

- You can draw five imaginary lines on either side of the centre line, going from head to toes and head to fingertips.
- If the stress or discomfort is on the side of the body, it is zone 5, and if it is in the chest area, it can be any of the zones!

How to Reflex

- To be effective with our touch, we use a technique called thumb-walking, involving a combination of right force, pressure and support.
- Normal pressure for reflexing is the kind of pressure that you would use for crushing a ripe grape.

- Try this out with a grape that is ripe to get the feel of the pressure and get accustomed to it.
- Lighter pressure should be applied for infants, the very sick or weak, and the elderly.
- Lighter pressure must also be used for very sensitive persons.
- To play it safe, start with a light pressure, gradually increasing it.
- As you work the area, you can go deeper with your touch, watching carefully the responses of the patient as you reflex for him/her.
- Anybody can have tender spots on their feet, even the most healthy, and the aim of reflexing is to work

with the tenderness by applying appropriate pressure to it.

- Tender spots could be due to problems with the bones or old injuries, such as a wound or a sprain in the area, problems with a muscle or a tendon, or choking of energy between the reflex and the related area of the body.

- The best way of getting the thumb into action when you reflex is with a gliding, wave-like motion.

- Just like a caterpillar uses leverage from its body to push forward, similarly exert a little force from your shoulder area to the first joint of your thumb.

- This gentle force from the shoulder helps the thumb's first joint to move forward smoothly on the surface of the skin.
- With practice, you can slowly develop a rhythm with the wave-like action of your thumb.
- In order to rest your thumb, alternate between using each hand and its thumb.
- Be very careful that you do not ever jab at the foot with your thumb.

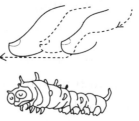

Caterpillar's Wave-like Movement with the Thumb

- Reflexing is micro-movements moving forward a little at a time, unlike a massage, which uses broader actions of hands.
- The skin of the first joint of the thumb should remain in contact with the body.
- If you find it difficult to move your thumb smoothly over the skin surface, you can use talcum powder, cream, oil or lotion on the skin.
- While reflexing, make use of one hand. Use the other hand to hold the foot in position.
- Remember that while you are using the thumb for reflexing, the

other fingers are supporting the thumb-work by providing a good grip on any part of the foot.

Reflexing a Foot

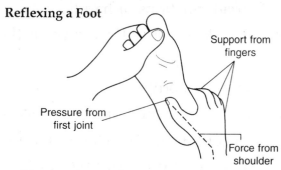

Support from fingers

Pressure from first joint

Force from shoulder

- If you have long nails, adjust the angle of your thumb to the reflex area accordingly. But it is best to have short nails for this purpose.

- When you are reflexing someone else's foot, do not use a commercial tool unless you already have a vast experience with reflexology.

- Also remember, do not ever reflex over broken skin, bruises, wounds or severe varicose veins.
- Only medical professionals are licensed to diagnose, while your object of reflexing is only to ease the stress in the body.
- It is very important to have a positive attitude towards touching, as important as the touch itself.
- Understanding how reflexology works is something quite difficult, but generally, how it functions can be studied from the diagram on the next page.
- When the brain receives a stress message from the affected colon

How Reflexology Works

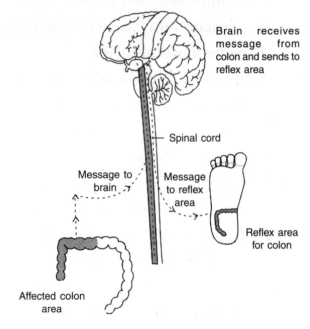

Brain receives message from colon and sends to reflex area

Spinal cord

Message to brain

Message to reflex area

Reflex area for colon

Affected colon area

region, it sends a response message to the reflex area.

- When the corresponding colon area on the foot is reflexed, the foot sends a message back to the brain, which in turn conveys it to the colon and the blockages of energy are lessened to promote balancing of energy.

- Body energy gets balanced by reflexing as pain is reduced or completely eliminated.
- The immune system gets stimulated, enabling the body to function naturally when reflexing takes place.
- When the feet are worked on deeply, or for more than 20 minutes, toxins may be released. Hence, plenty of water needs to be consumed to flush these out from the body.

- A tender reflex area suggests that extra attention needs to be given to that area on the foot.

- Continue reflexing on the tender spot till it becomes less tender.

- When you reflex on other people, make sure they are comfortable while you are working.

- With practise, you will be able to identify the tender area from the rest of the surrounding area.

- While you are reflexing on your own body, breathe in deeply and breathe out slowly.

- Each person may react differently to reflexing; some find it energising, while others find it relaxing.

Reflexing Areas of Feet and Hands

- In reflexology, nobody knows for sure how the connection is made between the feet and the body, for they are only theories. Only by experimenting on each individual will one know, from their reactions, the effects of reflexing.

- Though the body looks symmetrical and normal from outside, inside the body, things are very different, and hence, the reflex areas of the right sole may be different from those on the left.

- It is always wiser to reflex a broader area of the foot, since the stress in a particular area of the body may also be affecting a broader area.

Pituitary Gland

- The reflex area to the pituitary gland is found more or less in the centre of the fleshy pad of the big toe in both feet.
- It is also to be found in the centre of the fleshy pad of the thumb in both hands.

- By reflexing this area on the soles of the feet, the imbalance in the hormonal system is corrected. It also helps in alleviating fever and insomnia conditions.

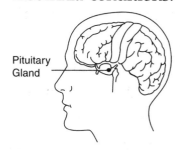

Pituitary Gland

Pituitary Gland Reflex
(shaded area should
also be reflexed)

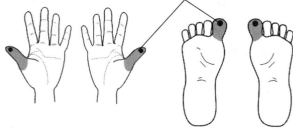

Head / Skull / Brain

- The reflex areas to the head and brain are found in the toes and a little below them.
- The areas in the hands are the fingertips, up to the first joint in the fingers.
- By reflexing corresponding areas on the toes and soles, damages to the brain, like Parkinson's disease, headaches, migraines, hearing or muscular problems, sight disorders, etc. can be set right to a certain extent, depending on their severity.

Spine and Back Muscles

- The reflex areas to the top of the
  spine are found on the inner edge
  of the big toes or thumbs.

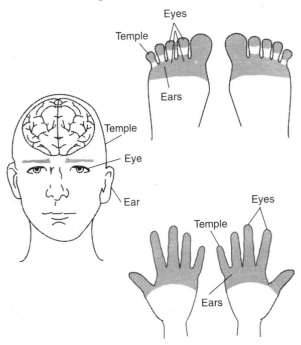

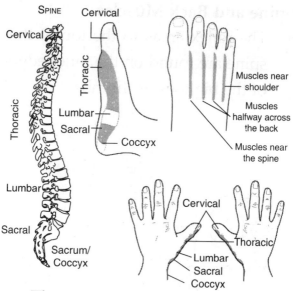

- The remaining reflex areas of the spine are found along the inner edge or medial side of the feet.

Face

- The reflex area to the face is found on the top of the big toes or thumbs.

40

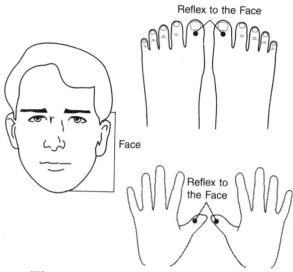

Reflex to the Face

Face

Reflex to the Face

- This area includes reflexes to eyes, nose, teeth, lips and muscles of the face.

- The right side of the face is represented on the right foot, and the left side of the face on the left foot.

Sinuses

- The reflex areas to the sinuses are found all the way up the second, third, fourth and fifth toes, and also up the sides of these toes or fingers.

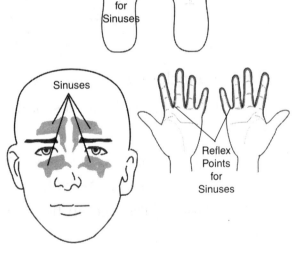

Reflex Points for Sinuses

Sinuses

Reflex Points for Sinuses

Shoulders

- The reflex area to the shoulders and their surrounding muscles is found around the base of the fifth toe on the sole of the foot or the fifth finger of the hand.

- The reflex area to the right shoulder is in the right foot or

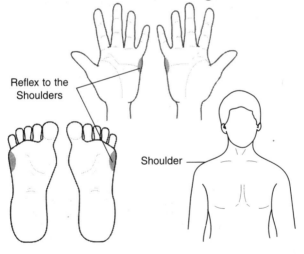

Reflex to the Shoulders

Shoulder

43

hand, and similarly, to the left
shoulder in the left foot or hand.

Upper and Lower Arm

- The reflex area to the upper arm is
found on the outer border, or
lateral side, of the foot or hand,
slightly towards the top, while the
reflex area to the lower arm is just

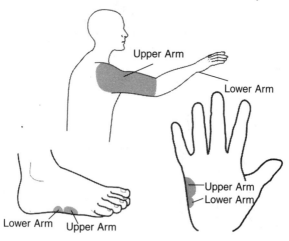

below the area that corresponds to the upper arm.

- The right arm will be represented by the right foot or hand, and the left arm by the left foot or hand.

Thyroid Gland

- The reflex area to the thyroid gland is found in the base of the big toe or the thumb.

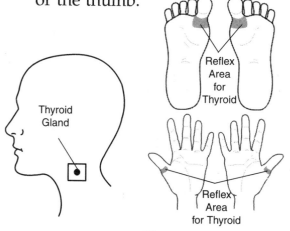

Parathyroid Glands

- The reflex area to the parathyroid glands is near those related to the thyroid gland.

- The upper parathyroid gland reflexes are found in the upper, lateral region of the thyroid reflex region, that lies in the upper part of the ball of the big toe or thumb.

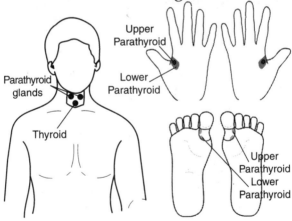

- The lower parathyroid reflex areas are found in the lower, lateral margins of the thyroid reflex areas on the feet and hands.

Lungs
- The reflex area to the lungs is found in the centre of the ball of each foot.

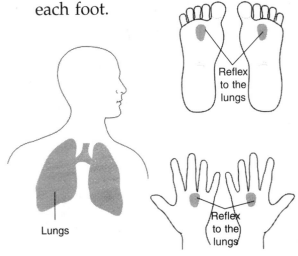

Reflex to the lungs

Lungs

Reflex to the lungs

47

- The reflex area of the right lung is found in the right foot or hand, and that of the left lung in the left foot or hand.

Trachea and Bronchi

The reflex areas to the trachea (windpipe) and the bronchi are on the medial side, at the base of the big toe or thumb, and across, into the lung reflex area.

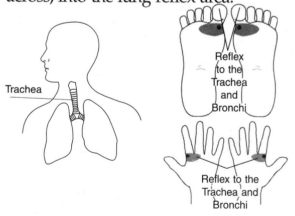

Trachea

Reflex to the Trachea and Bronchi

Reflex to the Trachea and Bronchi

48

Sternum and Ribs

- The reflex area to the sternum is found on the top of the foot, just below the base of the big toe, or thumb on the medial side.

- The reflex area to the ribs is found in both feet or hands, across the width, below the toes or fingers.

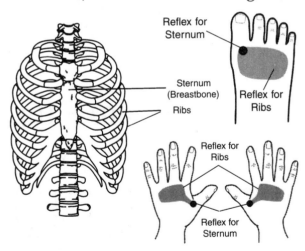

Reflex for Sternum

Sternum (Breastbone)

Ribs

Reflex for Ribs

Reflex for Ribs

Reflex for Sternum

Diaphragm

- The reflex area to the diaphragm is found in both feet and hands. It lies just below the ball of the big toe or the thumb.

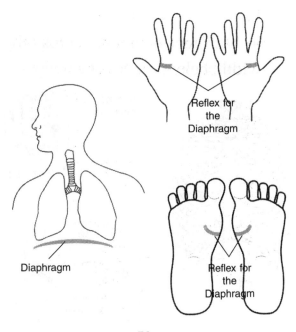

Reflex for
the
Diaphragm

Diaphragm

Reflex for
the
Diaphragm

Solar Plexus

- The reflex area to the solar plexus
  is found just below the reflex area
  for the diaphragm, where it ends
  in the middle of the foot or hand.

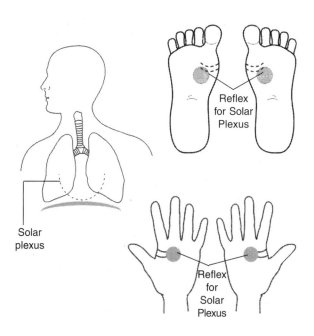

Solar
plexus

Reflex
for Solar
Plexus

Reflex
for
Solar
Plexus

Heart

- The reflex area to the heart lies just above that for the diaphragm, i.e. in the ball at the base of the big toe, or at the base of the index finger.

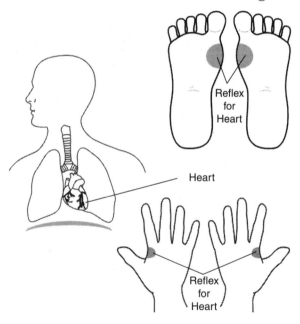

Reflex for Heart

Heart

Reflex for Heart

Thymus

- The reflex area to the thymus is found just above the area for the heart, and at the base of the big toe or thumb.

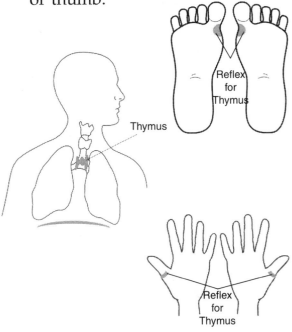

Thymus

Reflex for Thymus

Reflex for Thymus

Liver

- The reflex area to the liver is found on the sole of the right foot or palm of the right hand, covering a wide area stretching from the middle half of the foot or hand to just below the reflex area for the diaphragm.

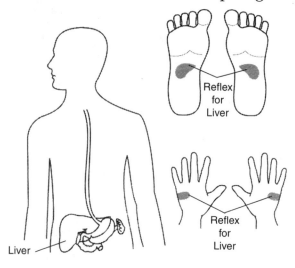

Reflex for Liver

Reflex for Liver

Liver

Gall Bladder

• The reflex area to the gall bladder
is in the sole of the right foot or
the palm of the right hand, exactly
in its centre.

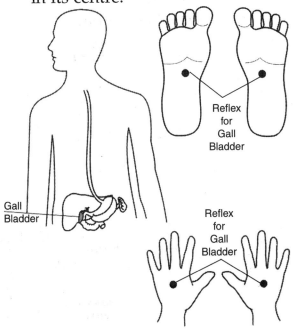

Reflex
for
Gall
Bladder

Gall
Bladder

Reflex
for
Gall
Bladder

Spleen

- The reflex area to the spleen is in the sole of the left foot or palm of the left hand, on the left side above an imaginary line that splits the foot horizontally in half.

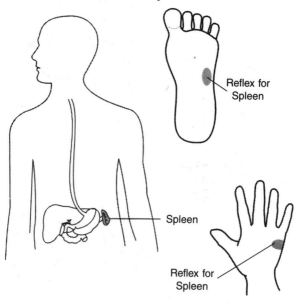

Reflex for Spleen

Spleen

Reflex for Spleen

Pancreas

- The reflex area to the pancreas is found in the soles of both feet or palms of both hands, just opposite the reflex areas for the spleen (on the left foot or hand).

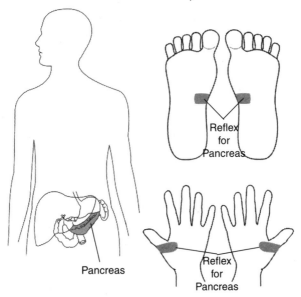

Reflex for Pancreas

Pancreas

Reflex for Pancreas

Stomach

- The reflex area to the stomach is found in both soles and palms, in the same location as the pancreas, but covering a wider area.

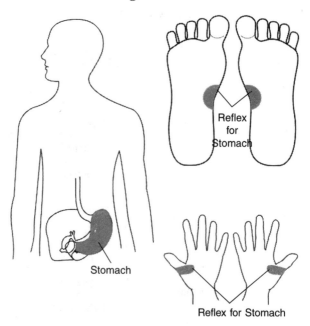

Stomach

Reflex for Stomach

Reflex for Stomach

Small and Large Intestines

- The reflex area to the small intestine is in the soles and palms, just below the reflex areas for the stomach.
- The reflex area to the large intestine, in the soles of both feet and palms of both hands, starts from above the area for the small intestine and continue to its sides.

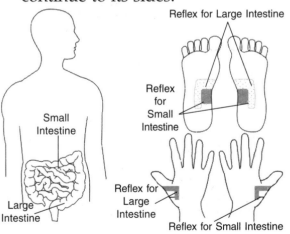

Reflex for Large Intestine

Reflex for Small Intestine

Small Intestine

Large Intestine

Reflex for Large Intestine

Reflex for Small Intestine

Appendix

- The reflex area to the appendix is found on the sole of the right foot or right palm, beside the reflex area of the large intestine, that is, to the side of the small intestine.

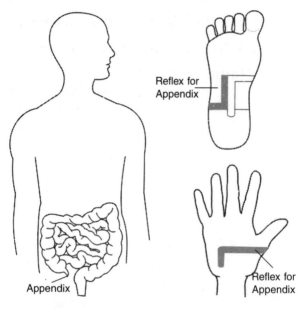

Reflex for Appendix

Appendix

Reflex for Appendix

Ileo-caecal valve

- The reflex area to the ileo-caecal valve is found on the sole of the right foot or right palm, beside the reflex area for the appendix.

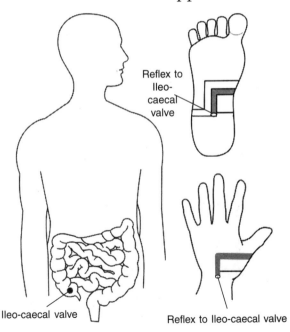

Reflex to Ileo-caecal valve

Ileo-caecal valve

Reflex to Ileo-caecal valve

Bladder

- The reflex area to the bladder is found on the medial sides of the foot, just below the reflex area of the small intestine.

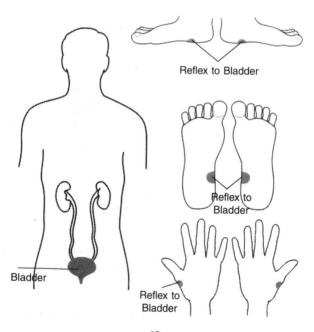

Reflex to Bladder

Reflex to Bladder

Bladder

Reflex to Bladder

Kidneys

- The reflex area to the kidneys is found in the soles of the feet or the palms of the hand, a little off the centre of the soles or the palms.

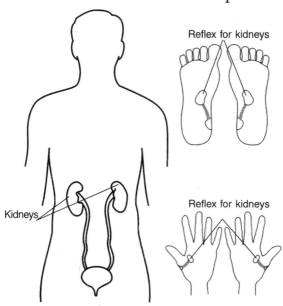

Reflex for kidneys

Kidneys

Reflex for kidneys

Ureters

- The reflex areas to the ureters are found in the soles of the feet or the palms of the hands, linking the reflex areas of the bladder and the kidneys.

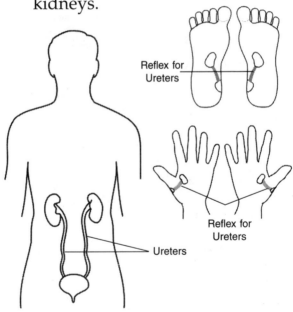

Reflex for Ureters

Reflex for Ureters

Ureters

Adrenal Glands

- The reflex area to the adrenal glands is the soles of the feet or the palms of the hands, just bordering the reflex area of the kidneys, above them.

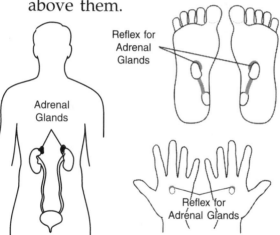

Reflex for Adrenal Glands

Adrenal Glands

Reflex for Adrenal Glands

Sciatic Nerves

- The reflex area to the sciatic nerves is found across the soles of both feet, one-third way down the pad of the heel or across the palms of both hands, continuing across the sides of the foot, below the ankle-bones and then up the back of the leg on either side of the Achilles' tendon, or in the hands, across the wrists.

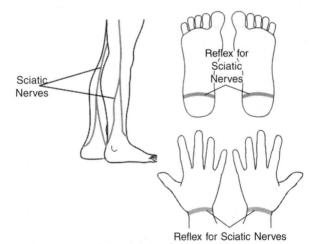

Sciatic Nerves

Reflex for Sciatic Nerves

Reflex for Sciatic Nerves

Knees

- The reflex area to the knees is found on the outer border of both feet or hands, very near the heel or wrist.

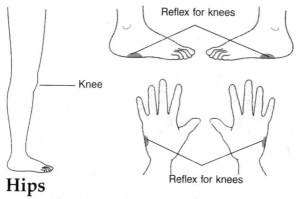

Reflex for knees

Knee

Reflex for knees

Hips

- The reflex area to the hip joints is found on the outer side of both feet or hands, in a half-moon shape, leading back from the knee reflex area to the back of the heel or the wrist.

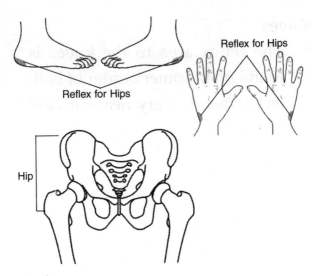

Reflex for Hips

Reflex for Hips

Hip

Ovaries and Testes

- The reflex area to the ovaries and testes is found on the outer side of the foot, midway between the outer ankle-bone and the heel, or on the outer side of the back of the hand, just above the wrist.

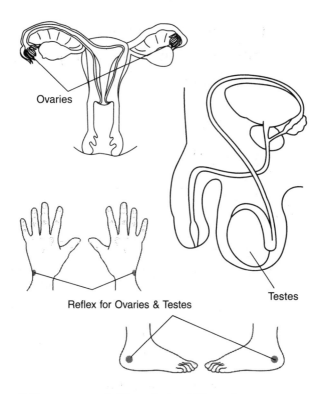

Ovaries

Testes

Reflex for Ovaries & Testes

Uterus and Prostate Gland

- The reflex area to the uterus and prostate gland is found on the inner side of the feet or hands, corresponding to the ovaries and testes on the outer side.

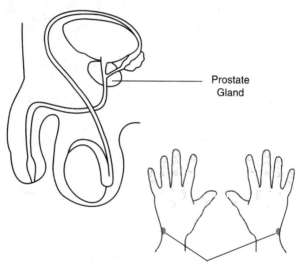

Prostate Gland

Reflex for Uterus & Prostate Gland

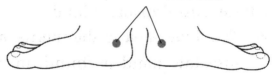

Fallopian Tubes

- The reflex area to the fallopian tubes is across the top of the foot, or the back of the hand, linking the reflex areas of the ovaries/testes and uterus/prostate gland.

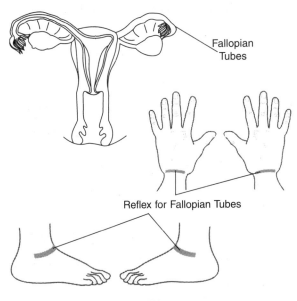

Fallopian Tubes

Reflex for Fallopian Tubes

71

Lymphatic System

- The reflex areas to the lymphatic system are on the top of the feet or the back of the hands.

- These reflex areas are treated from the web of the toes, down towards the ankle-bones and around each of them, or from the web of fingers, down towards the wrist and over its bones.

- The reflex areas to the upper lymph nodes are on top of the feet or hands, just below the web, between the toes or fingers.

- The reflex area to the lymph drainages lies between the big toe and the second toe, or the thumb and the index finger.

- The reflex area to the lymph nodes of the axilla (armpit) is found just below the reflex area for the shoulder, on the top of the foot or hand.
- The reflex area to the lymphatics of the breast is found across the top of the feet or hands, just below the toes or fingers.
- The reflex area to the lymphatics to the abdomen lies on the top of the feet or hands, right in the centre.
- The reflex areas to the lymphatics of the pelvis and groin are on the top of the feet, between the ankle-bones and around the inner and outer ankle-bones, or across the back of the wrist.

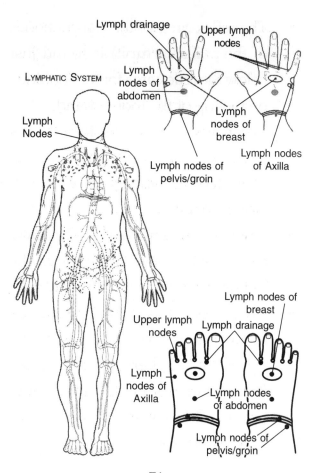

LYMPHATIC SYSTEM

Lymph drainage

Upper lymph nodes

Lymph nodes of abdomen

Lymph nodes of breast

Lymph nodes of Axilla

Lymph Nodes

Lymph nodes of pelvis/groin

Lymph nodes of breast

Upper lymph nodes

Lymph drainage

Lymph nodes of Axilla

Lymph nodes of abdomen

Lymph nodes of pelvis/groin

74

Teeth

- The reflexes to the teeth are found on the top of the feet, in the centre of each toe, or on the top of the hands in each finger, just above the web.

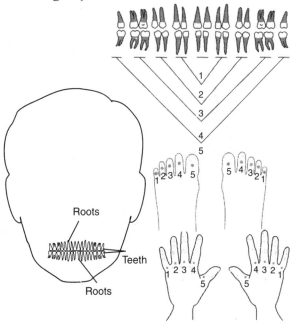

Neck

- The reflexes to the neck are found in the big toe at its base and in the thumb, correspondingly.

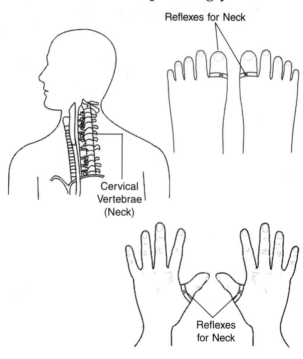

Reflexes for Neck

Cervical
Vertebrae
(Neck)

Reflexes
for Neck

Treatment of Disorders

Acne

- Acne is an inflammation of the oil glands just beneath the surface of the skin, causing pimples, blackheads, whiteheads, and in extreme cases, infected cysts and scarred skin.
- This is a disorder that usually starts during puberty.
- The reflex areas directly related to the condition include the face, neck, back, chest and the pituitary glands, thyroid glands, adrenal glands, reproductive and digestive

areas, solar plexus, kidneys and upper lymphatic areas.

Allergies

- An allergy is a reaction, such as a running nose, rash or difficulty in breathing, that occurs in people sensitive to certain substances.

- Common kinds of allergies are hay fever, hives, eczema, bronchial asthma, food allergy and contact dermatitis.

- The direct reflex areas are the digestive and respiratory areas, and the skin, while the associated reflex areas are the adrenal glands, solar plexus and spleen.

Angina

- Any type of spasmodic pain is called angina.
- Sometimes the spasms of angina produce a feeling of suffocation.
- Angina pectoris is a painful symptom of a heart disorder – a pain in the chest, which usually occurs when there is an unusual demand for blood in the heart muscle, but the coronary arteries cannot supply enough.
- The direct reflex area is the heart, while the associated reflex areas for these are the solar plexus, adrenals, shoulder and arm (if there is pain in these areas).

Anorexia Nervosa

- This is a condition, found mostly in adolescent girls, in which the patient eats little or no food, for psychological reasons, which, if not cured soon, might eventually lead to death.

- The main reflex area is the stomach, while the related reflex areas may include the solar plexus, pituitary, thyroid and adrenal glands, and the reproductive area.

Arthritis

- Arthritis is a general term for any condition in which the joints are the major sites of rheumatic disease.

- Arthritis includes osteoarthritis, rheumatoid arthritis, gout and rheumatic fever.
- While osteoarthritis may cause stiffness, pain and difficulty in getting about, whereby the hips, knees, fingers and spine get affected, rheumatoid arthritis is much more serious, with joints swollen and painful due to inflammation of the joint linings.
- The direct reflex areas are the affected joints, and direct massage for zone-related area of the body — elbow for knee, shoulder for hip, toes for fingers, etc.
- The associated reflex areas are the parathyroid and adrenal glands,

solar plexus, kidneys and pituitary gland.

Asthma

- This is a disorder of the bronchial tubes, causing difficulty in breathing.
- In chronic attacks, the consequences can be serious, if they remain untreated.
- Asthma is caused either by an allergic reaction that is usually inherited, or by an infection of the nose, sinuses, bronchi or lungs.
- The main reflex areas are the lungs and bronchi, and may include the solar plexus, diaphragm, adrenals, heart, spine, pituitary gland and the digestive area.

Backache

- A backache can be due to a strain, bad posture, a slipped disc, or even lumbago.
- A kidney disorder or gall bladder infection could also be to blame.
- Pregnancy also may cause backache.
- The areas directly affected are the spine and the neck.
- The reflex points, apart from the spine and neck, are the adrenals, solar plexus and areas having spinal nerves.

Bell's Palsy

- This is a paralysis in muscles of the face, caused by a disorder of the facial nerve (named after the physiologist Charles Bell).

- In most cases, it usually clears up, but in a few cases, the nerve is permanently affected and the paralysis persists.
- The face, head and brain are the main reflex areas, while adrenals, solar plexus and upper spine may be included for better effect.

Breast Cysts

- Most cysts of the breast are found in connection with the disease mastitis, and they are, generally, a harmless growth.
- The reflex areas are the breast, lymphatic areas, especially the axillary nodes.

Bronchitis

- Strictly speaking, this is an inflammation of the bronchial tubes, but often much more is involved.

- The infection affects the air passages of the nose, throat, larynx and the bronchioles in the lungs.

- In its worst form, bronchitis may lead to pneumonia.

- The reflex areas are the bronchi, lungs, throat, lymphatic areas, spine, adrenals, solar plexus, and if there is fever, then the pituitary gland, too.

Bursitis

- This is a painful inflammation of the bursa, which is a small fluid-filled sac, found either between muscles, between a tendon and a bone, or between the skin and a bone.

- An accumulation of an abnormal amount of fluid leads to the bursal sac becoming swollen.

- Bursitis over the knees, also known as Housemaid's Knee, results from the strain and pressure of much kneeling on hard floors.

- People who work all day with their elbows on a desk may get bursitis over the elbow.

- Bursitis of the big toe (bunion) is associated with chronic irritation in the affected joint.
- The reflex areas are the affected areas, plus the adrenals, parathyroids and solar plexus.

Cancer

- Cancer is any one of the several diseases that result when the process of cell division, by which tissues normally grow and renew themselves, gets out of control and leads to the development of malignant cells.
- These cancer cells multiply in an uncoordinated way, independent of normal growth-control mechanisms, to form a tumour.

- Cells from the original or primary cancer site may travel by means of the bloodstream or lymph vessels, to form a secondary cancer site elsewhere in the body.
- Cancer can affect almost any part of the body — blood (leukaemia), skin or mucous membranes (carcinoma), or bone and muscle (sarcoma).
- The reflex areas are the areas affected, and also the spleen and the lymphatic system.

Catarrh

- Catarrh is a condition in which there is inflammation and discharge of fluid from a mucous membrane, especially in the nose and throat.

- The reflex areas are the nose, sinuses, head, eyes, upper lymph nodes and the digestive areas.

Chilblain

- This is a local reddening, swelling and itching condition accompanying poor blood circulation, often caused by exposure to cold.
- A chilblain can occur on the fingers, toes, ears or nose.
- The reflex areas are the affected parts, adrenals, liver, and digestive and lymphatic systems.

Colitis

- This is an inflammation of the colon, the large intestine.
- The mucous colitis is a relatively mild ailment with little or no inflammation, a dull pain in the left side of the stomach, and diarrhoea and constipation alternately.
- Ulcerative colitis is a potentially serious disease, with marked redness in the colon, ulcers in the affected area, blood in the faeces, and severe diarrhoea.
- The main reflex area is the large intestine, but it can be widened to include the small intestine, rectum, adrenals and solar plexus as well.

Coma

- Coma is a state of deep unconsciousness from which a person cannot be awakened.
- Coma may be induced by some disease, poison, alcoholism, drugs or injury.
- Too much or too little insulin, in cases of diabetes, may also result in coma.
- A coma can become irretrievable, in which case the patient becomes passive like a vegetable.
- The reflex areas are the brain and the head.
- Extended areas may include the spine, heart, kidneys and pancreas.

Conjunctivitis

- This is inflammation of the conjunctiva, the membrane that lines the eyelids and covers the eyeball.
- Infectious conjunctivitis may be caused by various bacteria or viruses.
- The infection is highly contagious, being easily transmitted by hands or towels. Both eyes are invariably affected with swollen eyelids that tend to stick together, and a pus-containing discharge.
- The main reflex area is the eyes, while the subsidiary areas are the upper lymph nodes, kidneys, adrenals and upper spine.

Constipation

- This is difficulty in emptying the bowel, since the waste material has become compact and hard, making it painful to evacuate.

- Improper diet, nervous tension, insufficient exercise and routine use of laxatives may all contribute to the condition.

- The direct reflex area is the large intestine, while associated areas are the small intestine, adrenals, solar plexus, liver and lower spine.

Cough

- A cough is a protective reflex action, which tries to rid the windpipe or the bronchial tubes of anything that is blocking or irritating them.

- Inhaled dust, or an object such as a fruit pip, can even cause a bout of coughing.
- More often, mucus from the lungs or from the nasal passages irritates the windpipe and produces cough.
- A short, dry cough may also be brought on by going out in cold weather, influenza, or inflammation of the larynx, tonsils or trachea (windpipe).
- The main reflex area is the throat, with reflex areas of the bronchi, lungs and upper lymph nodes providing support.

Cramp

- This is any muscular pain, especially in the abdomen, where the muscle contracts and goes into a spasm.

- Cramps may occur in the muscles of the legs, especially after a prolonged, violent exercise, resulting in the build-up of lactic acid.

- Frequent cramps may be a symptom of poor blood circulation, often caused by diseased arteries.

- The reflex areas are the affected areas, as well as the parathyroid glands and the heart.

Cystitis

- Cystitis is an infection and inflammation of the urinary bladder.

- It may be caused by bacteria travelling from the kidneys or bloodstream into the bladder.

- · Cystitis can be acute or chronic, when there is the urge to pass urine frequently, accompanied by a burning, painful sensation, fever, chills and backache.

- Stones in the bladder or inflammation of the urethra may trigger the infection.

- The reflex area is the bladder, while the kidneys, ureters, adrenals, lymph nodes of pelvis, pituitary gland and prostate gland can add to the relief.

Deafness

- This is partial or total loss of hearing.
- In conductive deafness, something interferes with the passage of sound to the inner ear – maybe, a plug of wax, a boil, or a foreign body blocking the ear canal, perforation of the eardrum, fluid in the middle ear as a result of heavy cold or tonsillitis, abscess or inflammation in the middle ear, inflammation of the mastoid bone,

or overgrowth of one of the small bones in the middle ear.

- In perceptive deafness, there is damage or incomplete development in the inner ear, the actual organ of hearing.
- The reflex areas are the ears, with support from the sides of the head, upper spine, neck, sinuses, middle ear and solar plexus.

Depression

- Depression is a state of feeling dejected or dispirited, most likely occurring at critical or unsettled times in life.
- It can also set in after some illnesses, especially influenza.

- A depressed person, having a bleak, pessimistic outlook on his future, complains of constant fatigue or exhibits a variety of physical complaints, with difficulty in sleeping and fits of weeping.
- The reflex areas are ones relating to symptoms experienced, with related areas of the head, brain, pituitary, thyroid and adrenal glands, reproductive areas and solar plexus.

Dermatitis

- This is an inflammation of the skin, which can be caused by many factors.

- The parts of the skin affected are reflexed, correspondingly, on the feet or hands.
- The solar plexus, adrenals, liver, digestive areas and kidneys can also be reflexed.

Diabetes

- Diabetes mellitus is a disorder in which the body is unable to control the use of sugars as a source of energy, with insulin being insufficient.
- The patient passes large quantities of urine, is usually very thirsty, loses weight fast and lacks energy.
- Long-term complications may affect the eyes, kidneys, heart and legs.

- In severe diabetes, keto-acidoses, diabetic coma and death may result.
- Extreme care is necessary while reflexing to avoid the pancreas from producing more insulin.
- The major reflex area is the pancreas, supported by the liver, kidneys, eyes, adrenals and pituitary glands.

Diarrhoea

- This is a frequent and excessive discharge of watery material from the bowel, the danger being excessive loss of water.
- The cause may be unwise eating or drinking, allergic reaction,

food poisoning or various infections.

- The reflex area is the large intestine, while the associated areas are the liver, small intestines, solar plexus and adrenals.

Earache

- This is a pain in the ear, usually caused by an infection.
- A boil or abscess in the ear canal is extremely painful, and wax in the canal, too, can cause an earache.
- The main reflex area is the ears, and the complementary areas are the middle ear, upper lymph nodes, sides of head, neck and upper spine.

Eczema

- Eczema is a skin condition characterised by a red, itchy rash and blisters, where the skin often forms crusts and scales.

- These symptoms may appear on any part of the body and at any time of life, including infancy.

- It may occur if the skin is excessively oily or dry, or by repeated irritation caused due to use of domestic cleansers, alkalis or grease solvents.

- The reflex areas are the affected parts of the skin, with support from the solar plexus, adrenals, kidneys, digestive areas, liver and pituitary gland.

Emphysema

- This is a condition in which the air sacs of the lungs get enlarged and cause difficulty in breathing in severe cases.
- The cause could be exposure to polluted air in big industrial areas or due to heavy smoking.
- The main reflex areas are the lungs, with support from the adrenals, bronchi, solar plexus and the heart.

Epilepsy

- This is a disorder of the nervous system in which there may be periodic loss of consciousness, accompanied by convulsive seizures.

- The area to be reflexed is the brain; other areas include the solar plexus, spine, digestive areas and endocrine glands.

Eye Strain

- The eyes can become stressed by straining them too much.
- The chief symptoms are blurred vision, double vision, headache, watery eyes, as well as general soreness and bloodshot eyes.
- The eyes are the chief areas to be reflexed, while reflexing the solar plexus, adrenals, spine and kidneys provide added relief.

Fibroids

- A fibroid is a usually benign tumour that grows in the muscle fibres of the womb.

- Sometimes it enlarges to such an extent that it causes the womb to press against neighbouring organs, especially the bladder, and interfere with their normal functioning.

- Fibroid can also cause menstrual disturbances, such as pain, irregular periods and profuse bleeding. It can also interfere with, or prevent, pregnancy.

- The uterus is the reflex area for its treatment.

- Reflexing the ovaries, fallopian tubes, and pelvic and lymphatic areas also provides relief.

Fibrositis

- This is muscular pain, such as that of lumbago, wherein strained muscles go into spasm.
- The most common areas affected are the lower back, neck and shoulders.
- The areas to be reflexed are the ones affected, as well as the reflex areas of the solar plexus and adrenals.

Flatulence

- Flatulence is an uncomfortable accumulation of air or wind in the stomach or the intestines. The problem is eased by its passing out through the mouth or the anus.

- It can be caused due to too many aerated drinks, by the nervous habit of swallowing air, or by eating excess of gas-producing foods.

- The reflex area is the stomach or the large intestine, and the associated areas are the digestive areas, solar plexus, diaphragm and liver.

Frozen Shoulder

- This is caused by inflammation of the tendons, which produces stiffness and pain.

- The shoulders are the reflex areas for treatment, with the arm, neck, upper spine, adrenals and solar plexus providing added relief.

Gallstones

- These are pebble-like masses formed in the gall bladder, the specific cause not being known.
- There may be acute, intense pain if a gallstone passes through the bile-duct into the intestine.
- Sometimes, a gallstone becomes lodged in the bile-duct, blocking the flow of bile completely, resulting in the patient developing jaundice and serious inflammation of the gall bladder and the duct.

- The gall bladder is the main area for reflexing, with other areas being the bile-duct, small intestine, liver, solar plexus and adrenals.

Glaucoma

- Glaucoma is a disorder of the eyes caused by increased pressure of fluid within the eyeballs.
- If left untreated, it leads to blindness.
- In acute glaucoma, there may be considerable pain in the eye and the vision may become blurred. The patient often finds it difficult to see at the sides of his field of view and may see halos around electric lights.

- The area for treatment is the eyes, with help from the head, upper spine and kidneys.

Goitre

- Goitre is an abnormal enlargement of the thyroid gland, where the swelling is noticeable in the neck, at the front of the throat.
- It occurs when the body's demand for thyroid hormone increases but is not met, as sometimes happens in adolescence or pregnancy.
- The second type of goitre includes conditions in which the thyroid produces too much hormone, whereby metabolism speeds up enormously and the patient

becomes nervous, jumpy and overexcitable.

- The area of reflexion is the thyroid, with the pituitary, adrenals, reproductive areas and neck providing support.

Gout

- This is a disease in which the chemical processes in the body are upset, leading to the production of abnormally large amounts of uric acid.

- In an acute attack of gout, it is usually the big toe which becomes hot, swollen, red and very tender.

- Chronic gout affects the joints, eventually leading to severe deformities of the hands and feet, and occasionally, damage to the kidneys, leading to renal failure.
- The reflex areas are the ones affected, plus the adrenals, liver, parathyroids, pituitary and solar plexus.

Haemorrhoid

- This is an enlarged vein in the wall of the ano-rectal canal, the terminal part of the bowel.
- Also known as piles, haemorrhoid may bring discomfort or severe pain and may be accompanied by bleeding.

- The causes could be a pressure on the anal area due to constipation, or habitual or excessive use of laxatives.
- The rectum is the area for reflexing, with support from the intestines, heart and liver.

Hay Fever
- This is another term for allergic rhinitis or inflammation inside the nose due to an allergy.
- The mucous membranes in the eyelids and nose become swollen and irritated, and there is sneezing and a watery discharge from the eyes.

- Substances floating in the air, pollen dust, animal hair and household dust can all cause hay fever.
- The reflex areas are the sinuses, eyes, nose and throat, with further help from the adrenals, digestive areas and the head.

Headaches

- The blood vessels in the brain are interlaced with many nerves and it is in these nerves that the pain originates.
- Tension headaches are believed to occur due to emotional stress.
- In migraine headaches, there is an intense, throbbing pain in the front

and top part of the head, usually on one side only.

- Other headaches can be due to eye strain, common cold, hay fever and other allergies, high blood pressure, or injuries to the head, neck or spinal areas, lack of sleep, constipation, etc.
- The main area of reflexion is the head, and the associated areas are the eyes, liver, digestive area, neck, solar plexus and upper spine.

Heart Attack

- A heart attack can be caused by the blocking of a blood vessel by a blood clot formed in it.

- The reflex area is the heart, with more help from reflexing the adrenals, arms, digestive areas, shoulders and solar plexus.

Hepatitis

- This is inflammation of the liver, generally caused by a virus.
- Infectious virus of hepatitis is transmitted by food or drink contaminated with the virus, by a carrier.
- Serum hepatitis is transmitted by infected blood and its products, such as plasma, and by medical instruments, such as needles, etc.

- Starting with loss of appetite, fever and headache, it develops into jaundice.
- The liver is the main area for reflexing, while the other areas are the intestines, lymphatic areas, pituitary, spleen and stomach.

Hernia
- This is a condition in which there is a weakening of the tissue, generally muscle, surrounding an organ, and a portion of the organ bulges through that weak point.
- The most common sites are the groin, stomach, navel, brain and rectum.

- The reflex areas are the stomach, groin, large intestine and diaphragm, with wider reflexing of the adrenals, oesophagus and solar plexus.

Hypertension

- Hypertension is the state of high blood pressure, where the pressure of the blood is too high for the body's normal needs.
- It throws a strain on the heart, which has to pump harder to get the blood around the body, and gradually damaging the small blood vessels in the kidneys and the eyes.

- A cycle of events may develop in which the kidneys, damaged by high blood pressure, cause the pressure to rise even further.
- The cause for hypertension can be due to kidney ailments, arteriosclerosis, defects or disorders of the circulatory system or the brain, or tumours of the adrenal glands.
- The main reflex area is the heart, while the subsidiary areas are the adrenals, eyes, head, kidneys, lungs, neck, solar plexus and the spine.

Hypoglycaemia

- This is an abnormally low level of sugar in the blood, caused generally due to an excess of the hormone insulin.

- It may occur sometimes in case of diabetes due to an overdose of insulin injected.

- The lowering in concentration of blood sugar gives rise to confusion, sweating, anxiety, pallor, and eventually, loss of consciousness.

- Pancreas and liver are the main reflex areas, with the eyes, adrenals, head, brain and solar plexus being the associated reflex areas.

Hypotension

- This is the state of low blood pressure, which, in most cases, is not a feature of ill-health, as the patient's arteries do not harden as they grow older.

- In a few cases, low blood pressure is caused by malfunctioning of one or more endocrine glands, by circulatory trouble or by diseases of the central nervous system.

- The main reflex area is the heart, while the subsidiary areas are the adrenals, brain, head, kidneys and solar plexus.

Incontinence

- The inability to retain urin control bowel movements, or excessive indulgence in sex is called incontinence.

- This inability to retain urine may be to due to strong emotions or other causes, and leads to leakage of urine while laughing, coughing or any sudden movement.

- In women, this is usually the late result of strains to the pelvic muscles incurred in childbirth and happens at or after menopause.

- Primarily, the bladder must be reflexed, while supporting areas may include the kidneys, adrenals, pituitary, prostate, solar plexus and ureters.

Indigestion

- This means that the·stomach is upset or there is some disturbance in the digestive system.
- It may result in nausea, vomiting, excessive belching, a feeling of fullness or discomfort in the abdomen, cramps, constipation or diarrhoea.
- The stomach and the intestines are the main areas to be reflexed, with

additional support from the diaphragm and solar plexus.

Infertility

- Infertility is the inability to have children, maybe due to a disorder in the man or the woman, like sterility or impotence in case of the man, or an infection of the reproductive tract or emotional problems in the woman.

- The main areas to reflex are the fallopian tubes, prostate or ovaries, testes or uterus; other areas may include the lymphatic areas, and the pituitary and thyroid glands.

Insomnia

- Insomnia is the inability to fall asleep or sleep restfully, seen usually when a person worries that he does not get enough of it.

- Causes may be many – too soft or too hard a mattress, too many blankets on a warm night, overheated or too cold a room, too much light in the room, noisy outdoor activities, stimulating beverages, emotional or mental disorders, etc.

- The brain is the chief area of reflexion, while other areas to reflex are the solar plexus and the areas where physical pain occurs.

Jaundice

- This is not a disease in itself, rather a feature of a disorder, where the patient develops a yellowish skin, and the whites of the eyes may also become yellow.

- The reason for this discolouration is the presence of bilirubin, one of the constituents of bile, in the blood.

- The reasons could be an excessive breakdown of red blood cells, some disease of the liver itself – in which the liver cells are unable to deal with the bile in the normal way – or due to a blockage of the bile-duct.

- The liver and gall bladder have to be reflexed; for better results, also reflex the kidneys, lymphatic areas, pituitary gland, small intestine and spleen.

Kidney Stone

- This is a small mass of solid matter that has separated out of the urine to form a stone in the kidney.
- This may be caused due to raised concentration of calcium in the blood, kidney infections or other diseases.
- A stone may also block a ureter and prevent urine from leaving the kidney.

- The main reflex areas are the kidneys, with associated areas being the ureters, adrenals, bladder, lumbar, spine, lymphatic system, parathyroids and pituitary gland.

Knee Pain

- This may occur due to arthritis, damaged cartilage, pulled or damaged ligaments, putting too much weight on the knees (as in kneeling to scrub floors) or due to accumulation of fluid below the kneecap.
- The direct area of reflexion is the knees, while the adrenals, hip, parathyroids, solar plexus and

spine should be reflexed for added relief.

Lumbago

- This is a general term to describe the pain in the lower back, which is subject to a variety of strains, sprains and other disorders.
- Pain may be due to arthritis, pressure on nerve due to a slipped disc, strain or overweight.
- The spine is the main area to be reflexed, followed by the solar plexus and adrenals.

Mastitis

- This is inflammation of the breast, in which it becomes red and feels exceptionally sensitive or painful.

- It may be caused due to a hormonal imbalance or an infection.
- The breasts are the reflex areas, with support from the adrenals, arms and lymphatic areas.

Ménière's Disease

- This is a disease of the inner ear, due to which the patient feels extremely dizzy and nauseated, and may vomit.
- There is a constant ringing in the ear, accompanied by a headache, and as the sense of balance is disturbed, the patient has to lie down.

- It is thought to be a degenerative condition of the inner ear, which may gradually lead to deafness.
- The ears have to be reflexed first, followed by the head, upper spine, neck and pituitary gland.

Meningitis

- Meningitis is an inflammation of the meninges, the membranes covering the brain and spinal cord.
- It is a serious illness and is caused by bacterial infection.
- The brain and spine are the main areas to be reflexed, while the other areas include the head, lymphatic areas, pituitary and spleen.

Menopause

- This is the period during which menstruation becomes irregular and finally ceases.
- Most women complain of hot flushes, irritability, insomnia, dizziness and depression in this case.
- The areas of reflexion are the ovaries, fallopian tubes, uterus and pituitary gland, followed by the adrenals, digestive areas, ears, head and thyroid gland.

Migraine

- This is a disorder in which the patient has recurrent headaches, varying in intensity, frequency and length.

- Migraine attacks usually occur on one side of the head and are often associated with loss of appetite, nausea and vomiting, and in some cases, speech disorders or weakness.

- Classical migraine is associated with disturbances of vision, speech and mood.

- In common migraine, headache, nausea and vomiting occur, but there is no vision disturbance.

- The main reflex area is the head, with associated areas being the digestive areas, eyes, liver, neck, ovaries, spine, solar plexus, sinuses, pituitary and thyroid glands.

Multiple Nephritis

- This is an inflammation of the kidneys, which can be acute or chronic.

- The symptoms are headache, loss of appetite, nausea, a high temperature, puffy eyes and face, oedema in other parts of the body, and dark or cloudy urine – all this is caused by bacteria elsewhere in the body.

- The kidneys are the chief reflex areas, followed by the bladder, ureters, lower spine, lymphatic areas and pituitary gland.

Neuralgia

- This is severe pain along the course of a nerve or nerves, which may be caused due to an injury to the nerves or an irritation.
- The common types are facial neuralgia and sciatica.
- The reflex area is the face, followed by the brain, ears, eyes, head, solar plexus, teeth and upper spine.

Ovarian Cysts

- A common disorder of the ovaries is the presence of cysts – bladder-like growths containing liquid.

- Some ovarian cysts become very large, needing surgery.
- The ovaries are the primary reflex areas; other areas of reflexion are the fallopian tubes, uterus and lymphatic areas.

Paralysis
- Partial or complete loss of sensation or the power to move the muscles in part or parts of the body is called paralysis.
- It is usually caused by disease or injury to some part(s) of the nervous system, or sometimes a disorder of the muscles.
- The areas affected have to reflexed before reflexing the brain and spine.

Parkinson's Disease

- This is a chronic, slow, progressive disorder that affects that part of the brain which controls voluntary movement.

- Tremors, speech impairment, shuffling gait, fatigue and emotional stress are the main symptoms.

- Causes may be, in some cases, an immediate or long-delayed sequel of encephalitis (inflammation of the brain), or result of carbon monoxide poisoning, head injury, or arteriosclerosis in the brain.

- The brain and the areas affected have to be reflexed, followed by the adrenals, digestive areas, parathyroids and spine.

Phlebitis

- Phlebitis is an inflammation of a vein, often associated with thrombosis (presence of a blood clot in a vein).

- Usually, it occurs in overweight people who have poor circulatory conditions, such as varicose veins.

- In phlebitis, the area around the vein becomes red and painful, and in severe cases, there may be fever.

- The reflex areas are the ones affected, followed by the adrenals, heart, intestines and pituitary gland.

Pleurisy

- This is an inflammation of the pleura, the double membrane that covers each lung and lines the chest cavity.

- The symptoms of pleurisy are fever, coughing, shallow breathing and pain in the chest, while the two layers of the pleura become swollen, chafing against each other with every intake of breath, and causing intense, stabbing pain.

- The lungs are the areas to be reflexed, followed by the adrenals, ears, kidneys, lymphatic areas and shoulders.

Premenstrual Tension

- This is a mental and physical distress that occurs before the onset of menstruation.
- Nervousness, irritability, depression, frequent headaches, general oedema and pain in the breasts may occur.
- The reflex areas are those affected, plus the adrenals, fallopian tubes, pituitary gland, solar plexus, thyroid gland, uterus and ovaries.

Prostate Enlargement

- In many men, with age, there is a gradual enlargement of the prostate, an auxiliary male gland that surrounds the urethra where it joins the bladder.

- As the gland increases in size, it presses on the neck of the bladder, interfering with the proper discharge of urine.

- The main reflex area is the prostate gland, while the support areas are the bladder, kidneys, lymphatic areas and ureters.

Psoriasis

- This is a skin disease characterised by red, itchy patches that become covered with loose, silvery scales.

- The eruptions appear most often on the scalp, forearms, elbows, knees and legs, but may also occur on the chest, abdomen, back and soles of the feet.

- The reflex areas are the parts where the skin is affected, followed by reflexing the adrenals, kidneys, liver, digestive areas, pituitary gland and solar plexus.

Raynaud's Disease

- This is a disease of the arteries in the feet, hands, and occasionally, nose and ears, where the blood supply to these extremities is temporarily cut off, leading to numbness, followed by severe pain when the circulation is restored.

- The toes are the areas for reflexion, with support from the digestive areas, endocrine areas, heart, liver and kidneys.

Rheumatism

- This is a general term for a group of disorders which involve pain in the joints and bones, and the tissues supporting them.
- It may be due to rheumatoid arthritis, gout, osteoarthritis or rheumatic fever.
- The areas affected have to be reflexed primarily. Other areas of reflexion are the adrenal and the parathyroid glands.

Rhinitis

- Rhinitis is the inflammation of the mucous membranes lining the nose, causing a running nose.
- It may be caused by an allergic reaction, such as hay fever, but more often, is caused by a virus infection, such as common cold.
- The sinuses and nose are the main reflex areas, while the head, eyes, inner ear, spine and digestive areas are the supporting reflex areas.

Sciatica

- This is a severe pain in the sciatic nerve – the major nerve, which passes from the lower back into the legs. It is often associated with inflammation of the nerve or neuritis.

- Sciatica may result from a slipped disc or strain or injury to the lower back.

- The sciatic nerve and the area up and back of the leg are the main reflex areas, while the hip, knee, lower spine, muscles of the pelvis and sacro-iliac joint may be reflexed for better results.

Sclerosis

- Sclerosis is the hardening of tissues, a symptom found in a number of disorders.

- Multiple sclerosis is characterised by the development of hard areas in the nerves of the brain and spinal column.

- The main reflex areas are the head and spine, while the subsidiary areas are the bladder, ears, eyes, adrenals, lymphatic areas and solar plexus.

Shingles

- This is an inflammation along the course of a sensory nerve leading out from the spine, characterised by great pain and crops of small blisters.
- It may also affect people suffering from pneumonia, tuberculosis, Hodgkin's disease and other illnesses.

- The nerves affected are usually those on the abdomen and chest, on only one side of the body, sometimes also affecting the face.
- The area affected has to be reflexed; one may also reflex the lymphatic areas, solar plexus and spleen.

Sinusitis

- Sinusitis is the inflammation of the mucous membranes of one or more of the paranasal sinuses, the air-filled cavities in the bones of the head that connect with the nose.
- It often occurs during a cold, when the infection from the nose spreads

into the sinuses, or is caused by allergies, infected teeth or tonsils, irritation by cigarette smoke or dry, dusty air.

- There is headache if the frontal sinuses are involved, and pain in the cheekbones if the maxillary sinuses are inflamed.

- The sinuses and nose are the chief areas of reflexion, while the eyes, face, head, adrenals, neck, upper spine and upper lymph nodes are the supporting areas for reflexion.

Spondylitis

- This is inflammation of one or more of the vertebrae – the bones in the spine.

- It may be due to an injury or a disease, such as arthritis or tuberculosis.
- It is often a persistent, crippling condition leading to some degree of stiffness in the spinal joints and deformation.
- The main area to the reflexed is the spine, with support from the neck, shoulders, arms, solar plexus, adrenals, hips, sciatic, sacrōiliac joint and pelvic muscles.

Stroke

- Damage to the brain as a result of blockage or bleeding from a ruptured artery in the brain, causing a sudden loss of consciousness and paralysis of any one side of the body, is called a stroke.

- The conditions chiefly responsible for strokes are hypertension, arteriosclerosis and valvular disease of the heart.
- The causes are cerebral thrombosis, cerebral embolism and cerebral haemorrhage.
- The main reflex areas are the brain, head and areas affected, with support from the adrenals, heart and spine.

Tennis Elbow

- Tennis elbow, so called because the condition commonly affects a person after his first vigorous game of tennis, is the inflammation of the group of muscles of the forearm, attached to the bone on the outside of the elbow.

- There is pain in the elbow, resulting from excessive jarring and unaccustomed exercise.
- The elbow and knee have both to be reflexed, followed by reflexing of the arm, neck and shoulder.

Tenosynovitis

- This is an inflammation of the sheath surrounding a tendon, and of the tendon itself, leading to pain and stiffness.

- The ankle and toes are the chief areas for reflexion, while the reflex areas of the arm, neck, spine and adrenals provide support.

Thrombosis

- Blocking of a blood vessel by a blood clot which has formed in the vessel is called thrombosis.
- If thrombosis occurs in an artery leading to an arm or a leg, gangrene may result.
- Thrombosis in an artery of the brain, or in a neck artery leading to the brain, can cause a stroke.
- Thrombosis of the veins takes place most often in the legs and the pelvis, but it may also occur in the

portal vein that conveys blood to the liver.

- The area affected has to be reflexed, plus the heart and the digestive system.

Tinnitus

- This is the ringing sound or other noises in the ears, heard often due to a build-up of ear wax.

- It may also be a symptom of a disorder, such as Ménière's disease, otitis or other conditions that may result in deafness.

- The chief area for reflexion is the ears, followed by reflex areas of the sides of head, neck, solar plexus and the upper spine.

Tonsillitis

- This is inflammation of the tonsils, triggered maybe due to a minor throat infection or serious ones, like diphtheria, caused by germs.
- The throat and upper lymph nodes are the main reflex areas; the other areas are the ears, head, lymphatic areas, pituitary gland and spleen.

Toothache

- The most frequent cause of toothache is decay, which has penetrated the enamel and the dentine, the two outer layers of the tooth.

- The other causes may be an abscess, abnormal pressure from an incorrect bite, an impacted wisdom tooth or pain referred from somewhere else, such as neuralgia in a facial nerve.
- The teeth have to be reflexed, with support from the face and solar plexus.

Ulcers

- An ulcer is an inflamed, open sore on the skin or on the mucous membrane lining a body cavity.
- There are various types of ulcers – peptic, ulcerative colitis, mouth ulcers, syphilis, decubitus (bedsore) or skin cancer – affecting

the stomach, duodenum, colon, mouth, genitals and skin.

- The direct areas for reflexing are the affected areas, with support from the digestive areas and heart.

Varicose Veins

- This is an abnormally dilated and knotted blood vessel, fairly close to the surface of the skin, usually in the leg.
- The main cause is the weakening of the valves in the veins that are meant to prevent the blood from flowing backwards.
- The areas affected have to be reflexed, with support from the

abdominal areas, digestive areas
and heart.

Vertigo

- This is extreme dizziness in which
  the victim feels that either he is
  being whirled about in space or
  that things are whirling about him.
  It is accompanied by a feeling of
  nausea and vomiting.

- Vertigo may be caused due to
  Ménière's disease by a temporary
  reduction in the blood supply to
  the brain, hypertension,
  arteriosclerosis, or by taking
  certain drugs or too much
  consumption of alcohol.

- The ears are the main reflex areas, while the other areas are the head, inner ear, neck, sinuses, solar plexus and the upper spine.